"THOUGHTS"

"THOUGHTS"

24 Rhyming Reflections of HME and CFS/ME

Hereditary Multiple Exostoses and Chronic Fatigue Syndrome/Myalgic Encephalomyelitis

A selection of rhymes written to explore my thoughts and feelings when spoken words and the ability to express myself were just not enough.

8th Edition last updated November 2017

HELEN BEESTON

ISBN-13: 978-1499527360

i

Helen Beeston

DEDICATION

A very special thank you to

Vanessa for the initial suggestion that I should get it published.

Fran - who has pestered me (in the nicest possible way) since the New Year, to get writing and finish the book for publishing.

My other proof readers/advisers Matthew, Deborah, Kay, and Jackie.

Thank you to everyone else who has encouraged and supported me to publish this book, there are just too many of you to name.

DONATIONS

By buying this book you have helped to pay towards more research in to HME and CFS/ME

A further donation will be given if purchased via Amazon link in Let's do it for ME! www.ldifme.org

If you would like to give a further donation, please visit https://www.justgiving.com/fundraising/helen-beeston1

"THOUGHTS"

CONTENTS

"THOUGHTS"

"THOUGHTS"

Helen Beeston

To B
love from

[signature: Helen B]

Helen Beeston

Foreword

I am me!

I am a unique individual who has lots of hobbies and interests. I love to learn and discover new things. I enjoy the outdoor life and love to travel around GB and Europe.

Of course, I am not perfect – who is? But I do try to stay positive and look on the bright side which can be draining at times.

At time of publishing this 8th edition I have been celebrating my 50th birthday. I'm married to Simon and we have a son, Matthew.

People often do not notice that I have any problems. At a closer look there are plenty of scars for evidence. From the age of 11 to 23 I have had several operations at the Children's Hospital and the Royal Orthopaedic Hospital in Birmingham.

I have Hereditary Multiple Exostoses which causes my bones to grow outwards in lumps as well as growing normally. It is now in the 3rd generation of our family, my father being the first, my son the last. The HME gene is recessive and therefore has a 50% chance of being passed on. My sister is unaffected.

When these bony lumps caused restriction in joint movement/ became painful/or grew towards other bones then they had to be surgically removed. More information on HME is in this book.

I have more than a dozen scars on my body and the only parts that haven't seen the surgeon's knife are my spine, head, left foot and right arm!

I have a restricted range of movement in most joints and muscle weakness (particularly knees and left arm) from nerve damage because of surgery.

HME does cause me fatigue, due to the joints sometimes not being able to move in their predicted plane causing muscles to tire more easily.

Over the last decade I have also been diagnosed with Chronic Fatigue Syndrome/ME. The HME and the CFS/ME are not connected. I have just been unlucky. Although I do believe that the HME has made me strong and not a victim or a quitter. I feel that in a way it has prepared me to cope with the debilitating symptoms of CFS/ME.

It is my mind that causes me more problems and holds me back far more than my body. I have always considered that surgery repaired my body physically; once the skin had healed it was the end of that episode. No one thought about the long term psychological difficulties. Fortunately, there is a more holistic approach these days than back in the 70's.
There were many emotions I experienced during treatment for HME. Unfortunately, but understandably, I chose to keep most of the feelings to myself and just took the experiences in my stride. Over the years the unprocessed feelings and emotions have been festering away and affecting my ability to function as I would like.

I have several phobias which I believe are a consequence of 'hospital experiences'. I decided to address the phobias because, although I was used to them, my personal space was excessive, and it was making it difficult to be near my family at times.

I received Cognitive Behavioural Therapy, this empowered me to explore my thoughts. I have always found expressing myself very, very difficult through writing and especially talking.

"THOUGHTS"

I have found that by writing in rhyme it is much easier to express myself. I feel it adds a sense of humour to an otherwise very difficult task.

I had a book very similar to this printed as a one off. I have shown it to many people and all have said how inspirational and helpful they have found it. It has been friends and family who have pestered me to get it published. I have selected 24 of my best rhymes for this book.

Most people can relate to the rhymes. You do not have to suffer from HME or ME.

Enjoy.

Helen Beeston

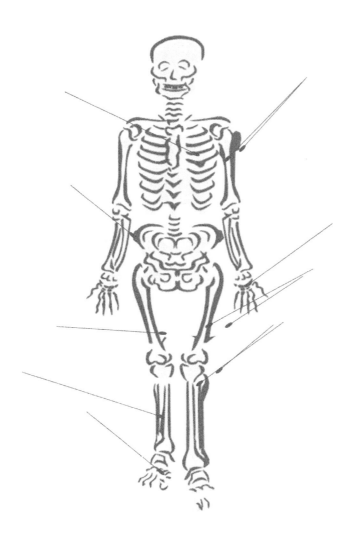

NB Arrows point to my bony exostoses.

My bones when I was about 12.

Note: Right leg 1-2 inches shorter than left.

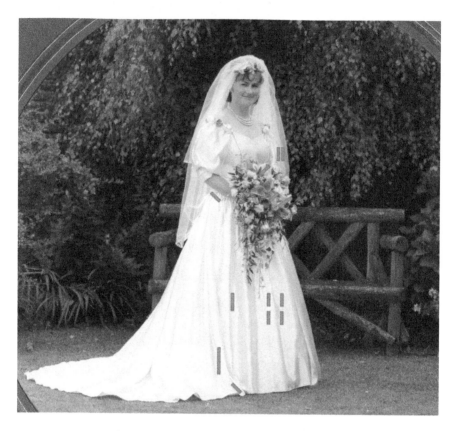

Me at 28, numerous exostoses removed. Scars to prove it!

2. Introductory Rhyme

I've written some poems.

All printed in a lovely book

You're welcome to take a look.

I've read some out

To explain what my story is about.

It's difficult to say how we feel

Our symptoms are so very real.

At times we look well

Even if under a horrible spell.

I am sure that you will relate

And identify a similar trait.

I hope my humour will make you smile

And not run a mile.

They may make you feel sad

"THOUGHTS"

But hopefully only a tad.

Have handy some tissues

In case it opens any issues.

I may give you a tool

If you use it, that's cool.

It's very difficult to start

It needs to come from the heart.

It helps me make sense of the thoughts in my head

It could make you sleep better in bed.

November 2012

3. Stay Positive

In May 2009 I volunteered to present my poems at a conference.

This rhyme was written to enforce a positive message at the end of my presentation.

I hope that it encouraged people to remember that HME is a very small part of the person. There is a lot, lot more to everyone. It is easy to look for blame when we are feeling upset, frustrated or anxious. HME is an obvious target. HME affects people differently.

"THOUGHTS"

Stay Positive

You may have funny bones

And you may creak and groan

It doesn't mean to say you have lots of moans!

Don't be scared

Try to be prepared

A problem halved is a problem shared.

It's ok to cry

Don't worry about showing feelings

And the embarrassment it may imply.

Others may not understand

But give them the opportunity to have a damn good try.

Don't hold back the tears

Or hide the fears.

Try to express the feelings

And explore the situation and dealings.

"THOUGHTS"

Don't be a victim

It's not that grim.

It will make it seem a whole lot worse

It doesn't have to be a curse.

May 2009

4. The Letter Has Come Through the Door OMG

This poem reflects my memories of waiting for the letter to drop through the door with the date of admission to hospital to have an operation which was not a familiar occurrence. My experiences were in the 1970/80's.

I have always considered that surgery repaired my body physically; once the skin had healed it was the end of that episode. No one thought about the long term psychological difficulties. Fortunately, there is a more holistic approach these days than back in the 70's.

The Letter Has Come Through the Door OMG

The letter has come through the door

It has landed on the floor.

It tells me to go to my hospital bed

This fills me with dread.

I have been there many times before

I know the score.

The operation has to be done

So the chance of getting out of it is none.

There will be a lack of personal space

Is that why it's such a frightening place?

The nurses smile,

When the doctors come I would like to run a mile.

They check that I am fit and well.

Draw an arrow on the bony lump

I am so tense it makes me jump.

They explain the facts

"THOUGHTS"

Say tomorrow no snacks.

They advise me to relax

And say it won't hurt.

I don't believe and stay alert

Feeling a sense of disconcert.

This fills me with sorrow

They say it will be removed tomorrow.

I'm in a familiar but strange place

An unsettling and restricted space.

An environment I don't want to embrace

Another scar to be added to the trophy case.

I'm playing clock patience

-Oh look I've got an ace.

I don't want the fourth king

And the end of the game it will bring.

It's how I was distracted

To limit the emotions impacted.

I clenched my fist

"THOUGHTS"

I am last on the list.

The day has come

I feel a strange sort of numb.

I'm so scared it's immense,

As if I'm watching from the other side of the fence.

Probably shock

From watching the clock.

Don't be frightened they say

I am, but I keep stum.

Have you eaten?

I reply not one crumb.

They check my wristband

To confirm I'm the one for the surgery planned.

I am wheeled down the corridor

Over the buffed and shiny floor.

They put a cannula in the back of my hand.

I try to understand

But all I can see is fuzzy

I will soon be dozy

"THOUGHTS"

I will hear them sat count to ten

I will be asleep by then.

It's all over; someone is trying to wake me up

And ask if I want a drink from a cup.

I am uncomfortable but not in pain

My muscles are under tremendous strain.

I feel as is I've been hit by a car

I feel like screaming, all because of a scar.

I really don't like the feeling of immobility

It seems to threaten my sanity.

I hate the feel

Sometimes it appears surreal

At the moment it is very real.

I feel so sick

My leg feels really heavy like a brick.

It's difficult to move

I know it will improve.

Until then I will be sore

"THOUGHTS"

A sensation I abhor.

To the highest degree

Dressings and sutures scare me.

The thought fills me with fear

It builds as removal time gets near.

It sends me into a panic

The reaction is gigantic.

My body and mind are at war

It makes it hurt so much more.

It is difficult to control

To relax would be the ideal goal.

The trauma makes me shake

My muscles hurt and ache.

I desperately want to escape the fear

Because it makes me feel so queer.

It's very unpleasant

And not going to improve at present.

It will take 3 weeks

"THOUGHTS"

To get back to my usual techniques.

Lots of exercises to do before then

They say do them 10 times and then do them again.

February 09

5. Sometimes it was Fun

Not all of it was bad, there were some good memories.

"THOUGHTS"

Sometimes it was Fun

When in hospital during Advent

Charity gave gifts to those with an ailment.

Sometimes it was fun

Ronald McDonald did come.

He gave me some felt pens

They lasted for ages and were used again and again.

Other people came such as football stars

It would have been helpful to know who they are.

Hospital radio was good

Requests would be played

The DJ's were voluntary and unpaid

I was always happy to hear my serenade.

The radio relieved the boredom

While feeling frustrated due to lack of freedom.

It distracted the ears from the constant buzz of noise

So many sounds -that really annoys.

"THOUGHTS"

There were advantages of being ill

It happened so often it became almost run of the mill.

I would receive many cards

Wishing me best regards.

Some relatives would come

Which helped stopped me feeling glum.

Bringing gifts such as Lucozade

Yuk! I haven't touched it for 3 decade.

I needed to absent from school

I certainly didn't consider that uncool!

I was always happy to miss PE

But missing science was bad for me.

I strangely enjoyed the change of routine

I considered it an adventure when I was a teen.

Even now after appointments

I enjoy a treat and a visit to Birmingham.

March 09

6. Asking for Help

This rhyme reflects how difficult it can be to ask for help.

I experienced a lot of tension as the person requiring the help, but unwilling to accept the support on offer.

I have experienced this from both sides and I know that as a helper, one can feel powerless.

"THOUGHTS"

Asking for Help

I want to ask for help

But what do I say

I'm not ok

I'm in a tizzy

But the nurses are always so busy.

Perhaps I won't ask for help

Tomorrow may be, but not today.

I want to ask for help

My pillows have slipped

My head is on the metal backrest

I don't want to be a pest

But I am getting stressed.

But the nurses are always so busy

Perhaps I won't ask for help

Tomorrow may be, but not today.

"THOUGHTS"

I want to ask for help

I want it now

I want to demand, but how

Without raising a brow?

But the nurses are always so busy

It makes me feel lousy

Perhaps I won't ask for help

Tomorrow may be, but not today.

I want to ask for support

I don't want to appear brave

It's just the way I've learnt to behave

I don't know the words to say

No words will come out, I dismay.

But people are always so busy

Perhaps I don't need help

Tomorrow may be, but not today.

I want to ask for help

I feel so lonely

"THOUGHTS"

But I am so aware that I'm not the one and only.

It is not just me

And that opening up more would be the key

Perhaps I should just count to three.

Perhaps I won't ask for help

Tomorrow may be, but not today.

I want to ask for help

Not to hide behind the smile

Appearing as brave as a crocodile

When people ask how I'm feeling

I want to reply without seething.

I don't want to say fine

Cause that's not the bottom line

But how can I tell people otherwise

To others my gestures, the opposite implies.

I want to ask for help

I have kept quiet for so long

I know this is so very wrong.

"THOUGHTS"

I am aware that I need to change

I'm frightened because that's going to be strange.

It's so difficult to know what to say

My behaviour has kept people at bay.

Perhaps I won't ask for help

Tomorrow may be, but not today.

March 09

7. Getting Better is so Hard

This rhyme is about the frustration of recovering from surgery. The body and the mind want to achieve different things. I often found it a huge irritation and let down when the brain realises that the body is not well enough to cooperate, and I found that I'm not as well as I thought.

"THOUGHTS"

Getting Better is so Hard

Before the op everything is so easy

It doesn't matter if I drop something

I can pick it up.

It doesn't matter if I need anything

cause I can walk to get the cup.

No exhaustion, to make me feel queasy

I don't notice the aching.

I don't realize how everything is so easy.

Now everything seems so difficult.

And even small steps seem huge

As if I have to do a somersault

With only a small safety net as refuge.

Whatever I need seems so far away

Even though it is close

I find reaching hard to my dismay

It feels hard to move a little just to smell a rose.

34

"THOUGHTS"

I have had an operation

I have a scar

Going out causes me a lot of frustration

It really seems quite bizarre.

Please don't knock me

Cos it will hurt.

I want to advertise my plea

But I don't want to blurt.

Shopping wasn't scary before

But now I am aware of lots of threats to my safety

So many menaces I can't ignore

It really raises my anxiety.

So many people

Going about their business

I am so scared I feel I may crumple

Challenging my senses and vigilance.

It is so exhausting

Both mentally and physically

"THOUGHTS"

I find it difficult adjusting

And need to do things very carefully.

I wish I had my arm in a sling

Or a plaster cast on my leg

To highlight the problem it would bring

And the notice that I beg.

Everything seems **so** so scary

There are so many noises

It makes me even more wary

And so many restrictions that that imposes.

My personal space is so huge

I don't want to let anything get close

I use it as my refuge

As if some sedative with a substantial dose.

I have recovered now

It's been over 3 weeks

I don't very often say OW!

I am beginning to forget the troughs and the peaks.

"THOUGHTS"

I am able to do most things by myself

And have rediscovered my independence

Now I am able to file this last experience on the bookshelf

Until the next time – and more endurance!

2009

8. Sadness

Even though I don't feel sorry for myself there was a lot of sadness which I couldn't explain. There were still lots of emotions that hadn't been expressed in my youth and these were holding me back from having fun.

I am pleased to say that these rhymes have been cathartic.

April 09

Sadness

Sadness is caused by many different things

I find it difficult to understand the feelings that it brings

The ranges of emotions are strange

I would love to have happier feelings in exchange.

Hospital was so different from home

Routine ticking away like a metronome

It was so diverse from the familiar

And in a strange way peculiar.

Hospital being the location

I remember the hugest sense of frustration

It was so scary

But I didn't know why.

There are so many noises

And the possibilities it poses

The talking, clunking, banging, groans and moans

That scared me to my bones.

"THOUGHTS"

Even today the sadness is still there

It hangs over me like a cloud of despair

I still don't understand the emotions

And I am scared and reluctant to explore the notions.

Steadily I will expose and understand

A lot of commitment it will command

It makes me angry and cross

The difficulty in finding happiness is a huge loss.

April 09

9. Doing Less

Keeping busy can hide a lot of problems. Sometimes time needs to be taken to slow down to enable the brain to process unprocessed thoughts. I associated doing less with recovery from surgery. I have had to challenge this and alter my way of thinking.

"THOUGHTS"

Doing Less

It may sound silly

And I feel a bit of a silly billy.

But doing less fills me with fear

The anxiety that invokes unfortunately is quite severe.

Slowing down gives me time to think

An experience that I fear could send me over the brink.

Thinking is something I try hard not to do

What am I scared of? – I wish I knew!

It should be easy to do nothing

And it should not feel depressing.

I am allowed a rest

After tidying my nest.

I shouldn't feel guilty

And perceive doing nothing as if I am faulty.

It is good to take time to myself

Without inconveniencing others or oneself.

"THOUGHTS"

Doing more feeds my avoidance behaviours

Developed subconsciously as my protectors.

I can forget and push thoughts and fears to the back of my mind

Where they can stay safely confined.

Doing more can prevent invasion of my personal space

And can keep people off my case.

I can keep my mind busy

I know its looks to others like I'm in a tizzy.

There are so many things that remind me of the pain of the past

The sights, sounds and smells are vast.

The change in routine

The potential events that are unpredictable and unseen.

The appointments and the enforced wait

Making me boil inside and becoming irate

I don't want to do less

As it will remind me of the distress.

April 2009

10. Why do I Persist in Feeling I'm Stupid?

This is the first rhyme that I wrote.

The following rhyme reflects my battle with myself to convince myself I am not stupid.

For whatever reason, I often consider most problems and difficulties as my fault.

This has been an ongoing issue for many years. I know it must improve, but it's very hard to change.

February 09

Why do I Persist in Thinking I'm Stupid?

Why do I think I'm stupid?

I'd like to be intrepid

But frightened of all things rapid.

It doesn't make me stupid.

Why do I think I'm a failure?

I feel so weak

When I try to speak.

I feel comfortable with a losing streak

Desperately needing to learn a new technique.

May be one day, I will have a winning streak!

It drives me mad

I feel so bad and sad.

How would I describe myself in a newspaper ad?

I would love to have the confidence to dress scantily clad!

That doesn't make me a failure.

"THOUGHTS"

Why do I think I'm daft?

The stress makes my body and head ache.

I can bake

I can make a good cake

I like to create and make

That proves I'm not saft.

Why do I think I'm stupid? I can teach

I can compose a good speech.

I try to give equal consideration to each,

I love nature and the copper beech.

That shows I'm not stupid.

Why do I think I'm not worthy?

I can be kind

I try to have empathy with all of mankind.

I am of sound mind.

I spend too long looking behind

Advice given from others to change so far declined.

That doesn't make me unworthy.

Why do I think I'm stupid?

I am alive

I can drive.

I occasionally take a nose dive

And shy away from a jive.

But that doesn't make me stupid.

Why do I think I can't do things?

I like to fulfil

I can learn a new skill.

I can pay the bills

I need to take pills.

But that doesn't mean I can't do things.

Why do I think I'm hopeless?

I love the hills

And take the thrills but get very annoyed with the spill.

I should take advice from people who try to instil

That doesn't mean I'm hopeless.

"THOUGHTS"

Why do I think I'm no good?

I love to travel

I don't live in a hovel.

Should I persist to unravel

The muddle in my mind?

I know I need to unwind

To communicate with mankind.

Does that make me no good?

I don't think so.

Why do I think I'm stupid?

I have enjoyed writing this rhyme

Making use of my spare time.

I must relax and stop watching the clock.

I can't keep running

And creating a block.

It's ageing my biological clock

It is best to take one step at a time

And to continue with the long climb.

Does that make me stupid?

11. Communication Is Scary

I find communicating with people very difficult. The reason isn't fully known but I'm aware that the cause is something much deeper inside me.

I have a real phobia about talking to people on the phone.

I can sit and ponder a task involving communicating for weeks and weeks.

It is very strange because others often consider that my communication skills are very good.

It's an anxiety that I so far have hidden very well and hasn't impacted too much until now!

I feel very inadequate.

It's so hard, I recognise the cycle that I am going through, but it doesn't make it any easier to break free from the cycle and to be proactive.

Communication Is Scary

My communication lets me down

And it makes me frown.

I don't like this scary place

It makes too many wrinkles on my face!

The words won't come out

What IS it all about?

My expression doesn't show the fear

It prevents people getting near.

I can convince myself that I'm right

But that only feeds the plight.

And I'm stuck here

Only me hearing my words in my ear.

Unable to explain how I feel

Thoughts going around like a wheel.

"THOUGHTS"

Unable to explain why I worry

And why my mind is always in a hurry.

Like I did while dealing with operations

I feel detached in stressful situations.

Hello, HELLO, I'm here

It's me, PLEASE notice me.

I'd love to be free

It's as if I'm looking out to sea.

November 11

12. I am Proud

This rhyme was a result of passing my 2 star for canoeing and kayaking. It was extremely hard work and I ended up with some tremendous bruises while completing self and assisted rescues.

There are other achievements that I really should be very proud of including earning my 1st Kyu for karate in July 2017, (next one Shodan Ho, provisional black belt!), over the last year I have completed my 1st year of a Uni course and working in 2nd year and how can I forget this book!

They are all achievements I believed were beyond my capabilities.

It just goes to show that other people have more faith in me than I do.

I am Proud!

I am incredibly proud

It's a very rare feeling

I want to shout it out loud.

It feels rather strange

But curiously appealing.

I do not allow myself to consider I have done well

Rather on mistakes and unfinished tasks I dwell.

It makes me sad to admit

That it's a terribly, terribly bad habit.

But now

I am incredibly proud.

It's a very rare feeling

I want to shout it out loud.

It feels rather eerie

But peculiarly appealing.

"THOUGHTS"

It does nothing for the soul

Preventing satisfaction and feeling whole.

There's always something lacking

Like a black cloud that's overhanging.

But now

I am incredibly proud

It's a very rare feeling

I want to shout it out loud.

It feels rather weird

But oddly appealing.

I have set my standards too high

And argued with many that it's not the case

Ferociously defending my need to deny.

Failure is not a concept I should embrace.

But now

I am incredibly proud

It's a very rare feeling

"THOUGHTS"

I want to shout it out loud.

It feels rather unusual

But funnily appealing.

Okay then, with what skills do I need to exchange?

I need to move forward and so how do I change?

It's easy to for me to say set my sights lower

The stress would be less and the anxieties fewer.

Therefore -

I should be incredibly proud

It shouldn't be a rare feeling

I need to shout it out loud.

It will feel rather strange

But it is actually quite appealing.

June 2010

13. Brave?

The following rhyme explores the meaning of brave.

Brave?

Someone said I was brave

I had to disagree.

I considered it was the way I had learned to behave

Any danger and I would flee.

I'd never considered I had been

But that thought needed to be challenged.

What does the word mean?

Who is the coward?

Before writing this poem

I considered it was me

I wanted to leave hospital and flee.

I was overwhelmed and felt overpowered

Because of an essential operation on my knee.

I didn't know about being empowered.

"THOUGHTS"

What is being brave?

What does it mean?

I had only considered being morally brave

That didn't fit my bill.

I never did anything

To fight opposition.

Just accepted the condition.

Who is brave?

The person holding the spider

The person up high in a glider?

The person who has rescued someone

The person who will tackle anything or anyone?

The person who has fought difficulty

Or is facing lots of uncertainty?

Who is the coward?

The person running away from the spider

"THOUGHTS"

The person staying on the ground, avoiding the flight?

The person who turns a blind eye

The person who cowers and hides to cry?

I would like to suggest

That the act of bravery is very much a personal quest.

A great test of inner strength from within

But it can be hard to know where to begin.

What seems brave to one

May make another act so as to not be outdone.

It's difficult to know whether the body is in fight or flight.

People need to give support rather than poke fun

It can be a big personal risk to reveal a plight.

July 09

14. Footsteps

Listening to footsteps around me gave an indication of any approaching dangers. Especially when in either hospital, attending appointments or being an inpatient.

I think that the sound can be quite scary and spooky.

"THOUGHTS"

Footsteps

Hearing footsteps can be scary,

They make me very wary.

Who do they belong to?

I wish I knew.

Clomp, Clomp, CLOMP, **CLOMP!**

While lying in my hospital bed

Contemplating eating sandwiches with nasty dry bread.

I listen and analyse the footsteps.

Who is in the shoes?

Where or who are they going to rendezvous?

Is it adult or child?

Smart and mild

Or maybe unkempt and wild?

Are they thin or fat?

Lazy or an acrobat?

"THOUGHTS"

Shuffle, shuffle, SHUFFLE ,**SHUFFLE!**

A lot can be presumed about the person

Thinking about it makes my fear worsen.

You can hear the definite brisk stride of a positive person

Could be professional, such as a consultant?

The uneven shuffling gait of an acquaintant.

The slow pace shuffle of someone in slippers

They feel so alien they could well be flippers!

The quick, short steps of a lady in high heels

May be pushing a trolley on wheels.

Creep, Creep, CREEP, **CREEP!**

How close will the footsteps come?

Not near me as a rule of thumb.

There are lots of people on a ward

They are likely to go the person who pulled the cord.

It worries me when people come close

To calm me the pill would need to be a good dose.

"THOUGHTS"

Thud, Thud, THUD, **THUD!**

Are these the footsteps that will come into my personal space?

When they get close can they see the fright in my face?

People near me make me nervous

I get angry with myself and self-conscious.

I am anticipating the pain

I know most of it's in my brain.

When I jump I get pain

It puts my body under of lot of strain.

A person touching me makes me jump

I feel so cross I could give me and them a thump.

They say relax and it won't hurt

Listen mate, I'm the expert!

One , Two, **One, Two,**

ONE, TWO , **ONE, TWO**

Knock, Knock, KNOCK**, KNOCK**

Clomp, Clomp, CLOMP, **CLOMP**

Shuffle, shuffle, SHUFFLE, **SHUFFLE**

"THOUGHTS"

Creep, Creep, CREEP, **CREEP**

Thud, Thud, THUD, **THUD**

July 09

15. Why am I Scared?

And

16. The Scared was Trapped Inside

In December 09 I found out that I would have to have a general anesthetic to have the procedure I needed. Nothing to do with bones this time, I was dealing with something very common!

I had been experiencing a lot of fatigue and just put it down to anemia and stress!

The following poems helped me to explore the thoughts prior to the procedure which took place in March 2010.

The emotional aspect of the experience really surprised me, I knew it would rekindle many thoughts and fears from the past. I really hadn't bargained on the huge physical impact it would have. It did help me to understand how and why certain sounds and lights cause me such distress.

I was expected to recover within a couple of days and return to work. Unfortunately, I didn't recover as expected and returned to work many months later.

It was now that the doctors started to take my constant fatigue seriously.

Why am I Scared?

I am forty-three

Not that old I agree.

I need a small operation

This is causing me a lot of frustration.

General anesthetics scare me.

I have had a few before

This may add to twenty-three

And won't be the last for evermore.

Am scared of the past or the present?

Trying to rationalize is torment.

The last operation was over 10 years ago

My mind seems like a yo yo.

I know I will go to sleep

And I won't wake up during the op

"THOUGHTS"

But it makes me weep

The shaking doesn't stop.

The thought of the bright lights of the room,

The horrible smell of its unique perfume.

Quiet sounds are so loud,

Sounding like a thunder cloud.

The past trauma is following me,

I feel so trapped, but want to be free.

My mind is distant as if I'm a castaway,

It's really tiring keeping scary thoughts at bay.

It will soon be over,

But it won't be a pushover.

I will be able to move on,

And what has to be done will be done.

March/April 10

16. The Scared was Trapped Inside

The scared was trapped inside

Waiting for the right conditions to coincide

Hidden from everybody, it couldn't escape

Putting me in quite a poor shape.

No one believed how scared I was

It was as if it was a secret

Kept close to my chest

My behaviour wouldn't show it.

I so wished it would

relating to the worry like it should.

I had coped with similar situations alone

No one to see my body groan

It was easier that way

Conveniently keeping everyone at bay.

"THOUGHTS"

Whenever I thought about it

Nothing seemed to fit

The pounding in my heart

Hidden, but just the start

The anxiety and restlessness

Sapped away at any cheerfulness.

They said I was scared because I thought I should be

I couldn't form an argument to disagree.

'There is nothing to worry about', they say

My feelings were then even harder to convey.

That doesn't make it easier

To understand the intense level of fear.

November 10

17. I Can't

I have spent most of my life trying to be not to be different or a 'victim'. Sometimes though I do feel as if this challenge gets a bit too much. I want to tell people why I can find things difficult.

I Can't

It's always a battle between the body and the mind

Sometimes the connection seems hard to find.

The mind seems willing

But the body doesn't want to do anything thrilling.

I know my joints are stiff and weak

Sometimes make me feel like a freak.

My torso is so stiff; I can touch my toes – as if!

People may think it's a fiddle,

It's not, I don't bend in the middle!

Do I want to feel hopeless?

No, because it causes too much stress.

I don't want to be the victim.

When I ask for help, it's not on a whim.

I don't want to be held back

"THOUGHTS"

Need people to recognize that there are skills I lack!

OK- my confidence can be low,

I need a bit of encouragement – I know.

It's not all bad, I can do lots of good things

And revel in the enjoyment that that brings.

It's just I think my reactions are slower

And my stamina can be lower.

2011

18. Pressure

The problems with my health and dealing with day to day pressures of work were seriously taking their toll.

"THOUGHTS"

Pressure

I have been described as emotional

OF COURSE I am

How much pressure can I take?

Before I SWEAR and say DAMN.

The demands keep coming

The thoughts become numbing.

Too little energy

Too little time.

Try my shoes,

I hope they won't fit.

They're not what I choose

I so want to quit.

I need to change my ways.

Find a way out of this maze

"THOUGHTS"

I need some understanding

to support a crash landing!

June 11

19. I am So Angry

There have been many conflicts and difficulties. I was aware that I had become very angry but not just at the immediate situation but something much deeper inside me.

The tests for my ongoing malaise showed nothing and I was finally diagnosed with CFS/ME.

"THOUGHTS"

I AM SO ANGRY

I am upset

I am frustrated

I am distressed

I AM SO ANGRY

SO SO **ANGRY**

SO SO **SO VERY ANGRY**

SO SO SO VERY VERY ANGRY.

Ok so you've the gist

And fortunately, not my fist.

I want to punch something hard

Ignore my ego – my bodyguard.

Something that doesn't answer back

So I don't receive a painful whack!

I want to shout and scream.

My reaction is too extreme.

Let me describe the source in words

"THOUGHTS"

It may ease the anger by thirds!

My body and mind have a lot of frustration

This stress has had a huge implication.

I haven't been well for a long time

Angry that I should be in my prime.

It has been so difficult to cope

I have descended a slippery slope

For the doctors I've been an intrigue

They tell me now I have chronic fatigue.

Even though it's only moderate

The impact on my life is great.

I can't walk far

I have to use a car.

I am too tired to drive

Making me feel less alive.

My muscles are stiff and ache

The restless sleep keeps me awake.

All lights seem so **so** bright

"THOUGHTS"

Adding to the discomfort of my plight.

Most sounds make my ears hurt

I wish my health would revert.

Is it real? I hear you say

The opinion has to sway.

Those who think it's nothing - haven't got a clue

You may have heard it called Yuppie Flu.

It drains the body

It drains the mind.

Like old batteries that won't recharge

Any energy saved will soon discharge.

I am an emotional wreck

What a state to be in. Oh Heck!

September 11

20. I am Living a Lie

The pressure of trying to be effective at home and work has come to a crisis point!

It all became too much, and I had made myself that ill and tired that I nearly fell asleep at the wheel while driving home from work.

This scared me and gave me a wakeup call; no job is worth ill health.

When I wrote this, I was very low and off sick from work.

When someone asked me why I was so upset, I just couldn't explain.

But then I decided that I was now living a lie. It was time for a reality check and to make my life more achievable to my health and stamina.

I am Living a Lie

I know that I am living a lie

I know I am deceiving your eye.

What is seen on the outside

Is not on the inside.

I have tried and tried

I need/want to hide.

I can't do things anymore

There isn't much to go for.

The me before has effectively died

I'm sorry that I've lied.

I am grieving for the health I had

I'm suffering really quite bad.

I've lost my way

The path looks grey.

I've lost my trust

Feel corroded like rust.

"THOUGHTS"

This makes me feel old and ill

Is there a pill to make me feel the thrill?

I do have something left of my skills.

I have to rely on my granny box of pills!

I so want to change

Which would be strange

To wake up and be well

And not to dwell.

Not to worry

Not to hurry.

For my mind to be calm

And relaxation be a balm.

December 11

"THOUGHTS"

21. Spoons

It was a life changing moment when I found I could explain to people just how much CFS /ME affects me.

The author wrote this to explain about lupus, but can be transferred to any illness or disability.

She explains to her friend that the spoons on the table represent the amount of energy she has for one day. Once she has used her energy up she cannot go and get any more, unlike her friend who can go and get more spoons from the drawer. When she gets to the last spoon in the evening she has the option of using that energy to eat or to have a shower.

See more at:
http://www.butyoudontlooksick.com/wpress/articles/written-by-christine/the-spoon-theory/#sthash.egQarzWy.dpuf

An excerpt taken from the story is below: -

'I explained that the difference in being sick and being healthy is having to make choices or to consciously think about things when the rest of the world doesn't have to. The healthy have the luxury of a life without choices, a gift most people take for granted. –

Most people start the day with unlimited amount of possibilities, and energy to do whatever they desire, especially young people. For the most part, they do not need to worry about the effects of their actions. So, for my explanation, I used spoons to convey this point. I wanted something for her to actually hold, for me to then take away, since most people who get sick feel a "loss" of a life they once knew. If I was in control of taking away the spoons, then she would know what it feels like to have someone or something else, in this case Lupus, being in control.'

"THOUGHTS"

Spoons

What do you see?

YOU see a simple spoon

To be used as a scoop

To get the food which you swoop.

I'll tell you what it means to me

A course that has altered since ME.

A path with debris strewn

A path from which I cannot flee.

How to use the last spoon

The right choice is a boon.

What option do I make?

Which course should I take?

I look ahead at an enormous maze

See the right solution in the distant haze.

"THOUGHTS"

How do I get there?

How will I fair?

I see energy diverted

Away from essential time

That could have been mine

To rest

To be at my best.

Energy to try

Energy to cry

Energy to speak

And not feel so weak.

Energy to walk

Without feeling vulnerable from a hawk

Not use a stick

And feel so damn sick.

Energy for fun

"THOUGHTS"

To be out in the sun.

To feel the rain on my back

To see muddy footprints on a track.

Energy to hear the birds sing

And appreciate the joy that they bring

To talk to a friend

And to accept the help that they send.

Energy to walk in a straight line

Before ingesting wine

Not to appear drunk

As a skunk.

Energy to keep up the fight

Energy to hold on tight.

Energy to fight germs and bugs,

Energy to give strength to others with hugs.

Energy to do something nice

"THOUGHTS"

Reduce brain fog and not to repeat twice

Energy to sit up straight

Energy to eat from my plate.

Energy to eat meat grazed on turf

Or from the food that swims in our surf.

Sugar is out of the question

Instead expensive protein powder in suspension!

No bread made from wheat.

No energy to digest a treat.

No energy to absorb nutrients from food

No energy to keep me in a good mood.

No energy to think

Fearing falling over the brink.

Response to be fast

And not the very last.

Time to sleep

"THOUGHTS"

And not end in a heap

Energy to see

Energy just to be me!

Energy to work and earn money

So serious the situation it's so not funny

My eligibility goes unseen

Any government benefits? -Not a bean!

Don't make me use the spoon which is last

Any valuable energy is consumed too fast.

No more spoons or energy available to me today

With costly and depressing fatigue, I will pay.

March 2013

22. ME Is My Friend

I consider that my ME was a safety valve. It made me stop and realise that things had just got to change.

"THOUGHTS"

ME is My Friend?

That's strange

Who needs friends like this?

It's because I need to change

If only it was that easy it would be bliss!

Tired, me? No, I'm too busy

So much to do, makes me dizzy

Germs take hold and are lingering longer

I do feel as if I should be stronger.

It's just because I can't sleep

Awake and counting far too many sheep

My concentration is not up to scratch

My memory is also an inferior match.

Why am I in so much pain?

Too much fog in my brain

"THOUGHTS"

Making it difficult to think

Body clock out of sync.

I didn't pass the test

So now - enforced rest

It has saved me from doing too much

Releasing the push from my clutch.

I should have listened long ago

Hind sight is great – I know

Again and again I'd been given the hint

Slow down and stop the sprint.

Now I have to listen to my body and my brain

Anticipate the impending activity and its energy drain

I can do things if I get it right

Get it wrong and the next few days aren't bright.

It's taking a long time to accept

Along the way, lots of tears I've wept.

"THOUGHTS"

At times it can seem tough which I'm facing

Essential need to concentrate on pacing.

March 2014

23. Brain Fog

Problems with concentration, thinking and memory ("brain fog") - reduced attention span, short-term memory problems, word-finding difficulties, inability to plan or organise thoughts, loss of concentration.

This is one of the most difficult aspects to live with, who would think that thinking could be such hard work?

I find food shopping particularly hard as it involved so many skills that ME can deprive us of.

I will often find that I have a large amount of food that we don't really need daily, i.e. baked beans, black pepper etc. but more important things are forgotten.

For more information go to:

http://www.nhs.uk/Conditions/Chronic-fatigue-syndrome/Pages/Symptoms.aspx

"THOUGHTS"

Brain Fog

Frustrated at not being able to think

Can send me over the brink.

Trying to function through a virtual soup

No good anymore to lead a group.

Brain doesn't work well

Planning doesn't gel.

Coordination feels slow

Previous skills and knowledge don't flow.

Watch a film and follow a plot

Throws my thinking into a knot

I try to read and extract information

Finding answers that need confirmation.

Random words are spoken

The thread of the conversation broken.

"THOUGHTS"

Incorrect comprehension is implied

Embarrassing! Now to curl up and hide.

Inability to plan

Reduced attention span.

Unable to think quick

Gives the impression that I'm thick.

Finding words can be tricky

My brain acts as if its sticky.

I need a calculator to perform a simple sum

Making me look as if I'm dumb.

This is so far from the truth

Ask me questions, be a sleuth.

I like others (with ME) are highly skilled people

Currently not at the top of their steeple!

April 14

24. Waiting for the Next Thing to Happen

I don't feel that this needs an introduction, the rhyme explains it all!

"THOUGHTS"

Waiting for the Next Thing to Happen

Lately life has been good

Better than I imagined it could.

It follows a run of events that were bad

That made me feel really sad.

I now find myself waiting

For the bubble to burst

And the fight to get worse.

November 13

It's been a year since things looked grim

The chance of the bubble bursting is now very slim.

I have more confidence now

And less of a frowning brow.

I am enjoying my new job

Less stress and doesn't make me sob.

"THOUGHTS"

My health is continuing to improve

I'm now not stuck in a groove.

I have less worry

No longer in such a hurry.

I have more time

To build to my prime.

May 14

The bubble has burst

I'm sensing the worst.

Very recently life has been good

Better than I imagined it could.

It follows a run of events that were very bad

and made me feel really, really sad.

When there is less worry

No need to hurry

Less rushing like a busy bee

My body decides to look after 'ME'

"THOUGHTS"

I've caught a virus, knocking me off my feet

Worry, made me white as a sheet.

This time recovery is quicker

Glimpses of better health flicker.

Fortunately; not crashed as low as before

Now time to rest and restore.

November 2017

25. What Keeps Me Going?

This rhyme was written as an introduction to me for my Facebook profile. I have added to it to portray the thoughts that are very important to me.

"THOUGHTS"

What Keeps Me Going?

I like to learn something new every day

I find it keeps the blues at bay.

It can be knowledge or a skill

Lightens the heart and creates a thrill!

I enjoy the simple things in life

Spending money can get me into too much strife!

I marvel in the colours of the rainbow

And the unspoilt whiteness of the snow.

I'm always grateful

Even when I'm feeling awful.

There's always someone worse off,

a thought not to scoff.

Whenever I am unwell, I try not to dwell

And look forward and not back

"THOUGHTS"

I know that every minute I feel like s**t

It's a minute closer to the end and getting fit.

March 14

"THOUGHTS"

Endnote

I would always remember the words to this song when times were difficult. I would often think it would be so nice not to have the issues that I was dealing with.

Often their grass isn't greener!

Wouldn't it be good to be in your shoes

Even if it was for just one day

And wouldn't it be good if we could wish ourselves away

Wouldn't it be good to be on your side

Grass is always greener over there

Wouldn't it be good if we could live without a care.

Nik Kershaw 1984

"THOUGHTS"

About Hereditary Multiple Exostoses

Taken from Wikipedia, the free encyclopedia
http://en.wikipedia.org/wiki/Hereditary_multiple_exostoses
(last edited 6 October 2017, at 16:57)

Hereditary multiple exostoses (HME) is a rare medical condition in which multiple bony spurs or lumps (also known as exostoses, or osteochondromas) develop on the bones of a child. HME is synonymous with Multiple Hereditary Exostoses, Diaphyseal Aclasis and lastly Multiple Osteochondromatosis, which is the preferred term used by the World Health Organization.

HME can cause a significant amount of pain to people of all ages.

HME is estimated to occur in 1 in 50,000 people

Pathophysiology

It is characterized by the growth of cartilage-capped benign bone tumours around areas of active bone growth, particularly the metaphysis of the long bones. HME can lead to the shortening and bowing of bones; affected individuals often have a short stature. Depending on their location the exostoses can cause the following problems: pain or numbness from nerve compression, vascular compromise, inequality of limb length, irritation of tendon and muscle, as well as a limited range of motion at the joints upon which they encroach. A person with HME has an increased risk of developing a rare form of bone cancer called chondrosarcoma as an adult. [citation

106

needed] Problems may be had in later life and these could include weak bones and nerve damage. [2][3][4] The reported rate of transformation ranges from as low as 0.57%[5] to as high as 8.3% of people with HME.[6]

Treatment

Surgical excision is performed when exostoses lead to growth disturbances or lead to disability. Knee osteotomies are associated with high incidence of peroneal nerve paralysis.[1]

Surgery, physical therapy and pain management are currently the only options available to HME patients, but success varies from patient to patient and many struggle with pain, fatigue and mobility problems throughout their lives. It is not uncommon for HME patients to undergo numerous surgical procedures throughout their lives to remove painful or deforming exostoses, correct limb length discrepancies or improve range of motion. Usually the treatment can be problematic. The osteochondromas can return in the same places and may be more painful

Genetics

HME is an autosomal dominant hereditary disorder. This means that a patient with HME has a 50% chance of transmitting this disorder to his or her children. Most individuals with HME have a parent who also has the condition. However, approximately 10% -20% of individuals with HME have the condition as a result of a spontaneous mutation and are thus the first person in their family to be affected.

HME has thus far been linked with mutations in three genes.

EXT1 which maps to chromosome 8q24.1[8]

EXT2 which maps to 11p13[9]

EXT3 which maps to the short arm of Chromosome 19 (though its exact location has yet to be precisely determined)[10]

Images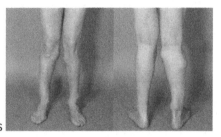

(I could have looked very similar without surgery!)

An Example Exostosis around knee joint.

http://radiopaedia.org/articles/osteochondroma

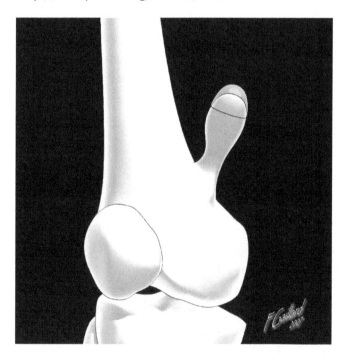

"THOUGHTS"

What is CFS/ME?

Taken from http://www.nhs.uk/Conditions/Chronic-fatigue-syndrome/Pages/Symptoms.aspx

CFS or ME?

There is some debate over whether the term Chronic Fatigue Syndrome (CFS) or Myalgic Encephalomyelitis (ME) should be used.

Chronic fatigue syndrome (CFS) is the term often used and preferred by doctors because there is little evidence of brain and spinal cord inflammation, as the term ME suggests. ME is also thought to be too specific to cover all the symptoms.

Myalgic encephalomyelitis (ME) is the term preferred by some people who feel that CFS is too general and does not reflect the severity and different types of fatigue. It also highlights the fact that fatigue is not the only symptom.

Chronic fatigue syndrome (CFS) causes persistent fatigue (exhaustion) that affects everyday life and doesn't go away with sleep or rest.

It is estimated that around 250,000 people in the UK have CFS.

ME is a long-term (chronic) fluctuating illness that causes symptoms affecting many body systems, more commonly the nervous and immune systems.

Many people with ME experience persistent fatigue or pain. However, ME is characterised by a range of additional symptoms.

Symptoms of chronic fatigue syndrome

The symptoms of chronic fatigue syndrome (CFS) vary from person to person and there are often periods when they are better or worse.

Most people with CFS describe this fatigue as overwhelming, and a different type of tiredness from what they have experienced before.

Exercising can make symptoms worse. This is called post-exertional malaise, or 'payback'. The effect of this is sometimes delayed – for example, if you were to play a game of sport, the resulting fatigue may not develop for a few hours afterwards, or even the next day.

Other symptoms

There are other common symptoms as well as fatigue, although most people do not have all of them. They include:

Muscular pain, joint pain and severe headaches

Poor short-term memory and concentration, and difficulty organising thoughts and finding the right words ('brain fog')

Painful lymph nodes (small glands of the immune system)

Stomach pain and other problems similar to irritable bowel syndrome, such as bloating, constipation, diarrhoea and nausea

Sore throat

Sleeping problems, such as insomnia and feeling that sleep is not refreshing

Sensitivity or intolerance to light, loud noise, alcohol and certain foods

Psychological difficulties, such as depression, irritability and panic attacks

Less common symptoms, such as dizziness, excess sweating, balance problems and difficulty controlling body temperature.

Authors comment; In my experience the NHS considers both conditions the same, The Hummingbirds' Foundation for M.E. has an interesting comparison chart for CFS/ME.

For more information http://www.hfme.org/comparisonchart.htm.

References

Christine Miserandino. (2010). The Spoon Theory. Available: http://www.butyoudontlooksick.com/wpress/articles/written-by-christine/the-spoon-theory/#sthash.egQarzWy.dpuf. Last accessed 9th November 2017

Dr Yuranga Weerakkody and Dr Frank Gaillard et al. (2005). Osteochondroma. Available: http://radiopaedia.org/articles/osteochondroma. Last accessed 9th November 2017

Nicholas David Kershaw. 'Wouldn't It Be Good'.by Nicholas David Kershaw. 1984. LP

NHS. (20/03/2013). Chronic fatigue syndrome. Available: http://www.nhs.uk/Conditions/Chronic-fatigue-syndrome/Pages/Symptoms.aspx. Last accessed 9th November 2017

Wiki. (2014). Hereditary multiple exostosis. Available: http://en.wikipedia.org/wiki/Hereditary_multiple_exostoses . Last accessed 9th November 2017.

Useful Websites

http://www.mheandme.com/BumpyBoneClub.html

Contact a Family: - http://www.cafamily.org.uk

http://en.wikipedia.org/wiki/Hereditary_multiple_exostoses

https://www.mherf.org/

http://www.meassociation.org.uk

http://www.actionforme.org.uk

http://www.butyoudontlooksick.com

The Hummingbirds' Foundation for M.E.
http://www.hfme.org/comparisonchart.htm

http://www.nhs.uk/Conditions/Chronic-fatigue-
syndrome/Pages/Symptoms.aspx.

Let's do it for ME http://www.ldifme.org

Useful Books

Ferguson, A (1985). Penguin Rhyming Dictionary. London: Penguin.
various pages.

Follow this book on:

"THOUGHTS"

  Helen Beeston @thoughtsbyhb

  https://www.facebook.com/thoughtsbyhelenbeeston

  Author Page

 Helen Beeston

"THOUGHTS"

ABOUT THE AUTHOR

"Helen was born and raised in South Birmingham. She moved to Wolverhampton in the Black Country where she met her husband. She began her career in Walsall training as a Registered Nurse for the Mentally Handicapped in late 80's and has continued to work in Walsall in different roles with adults and children with a learning disability.

She lives with her husband and son.

Helen was born with Hereditary Multiple Exostosis and endured many operations for HME from age 11 to 22. She was treated at Birmingham Children's Hospital and later the Royal Orthopaedic. Helen has had ME (Myalgic Encephalomyelitis) since 2000 although it wasn't diagnosed until a few years ago after she didn't recover from a simple operation and an infection.

Helen's cup always appears half full. Rarely is the half empty ever divulged to others. The smile hides so much.

Using rhyme has become a cathartic way for Helen to explore and explain her difficulties to others. Helen has shown some of her rhymes to friends and they have encouraged her to publish. They could identify with the issues, despite not suffering from either HME or ME themselves.

Despite her physical limitations, she has a zest for gaining knowledge. She loves to help others. She tries to lead a busy life. Some favourite activities include - enjoying being out in the countryside, exploring industrial heritage and improving her karate.

"THOUGHTS"

This is her first published book, but she has more ideas for at least another book.'

Made in the USA
Columbia, SC
18 August 2018